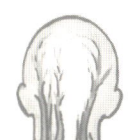

Published by Bryan Edwards Publishing Company, Inc.
Produced by Bryan E. Nash
Written and Illustrated by Flash Anatomy, Inc,.
Anatomical Illustrations and Research by Merideth Hardgrave
Edited and Verified by Thomas Braem, M.S. Physiologist

1994 Bryan Edwards, A Publishing Company, Inc.
All rights reserved.
Printed in the United States of America
No part of this publication may be reproduced or
distributed in any form or by any means or stored
in a data base or retrieval system,
without the prior written permission of the publisher.

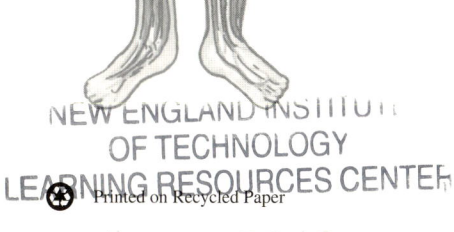

Printed on Recycled Paper

Lymph System
L_1

I. **Consists of:**
1. Extensive capillary network which collects lymph.

2. Collecting vessels.

3. Lymphoid Tissues:
    A. Lymph Nodes
    B. Spleen
    C. Thymus
    D. Tonsils
    E. Appendix
    F. Peyer's patches (GALT)
    G. Bone Marrow

II. **Function:**
1. Lymph drains though the lymphatic system taking with it debris, cellular waste and bacteria.

2. Lymphatic vessels serve as routes for lymph to be returned to general circulation.

3. Lymphoid tissues store, process, or produce.

4. Lymphocytes[1] remove the debris, cellular waste and bacteria by the process of phagocytosis. Through "immunological memory" lymphocytes can recognize previous antigens and fight them with specially created antibodies[2].

5. The ability of the organs of the lymphatic system to destroy invading bacteria, and remove dead and damaged tissue, make them essential to the body's immune system.

6. The lymph system also transports fat-soluble nutrients from the digestive tract[3] to the blood.

Cross-Reference			Definitions
Volume	Chapter		1. Lymph: Fluid collected by the lymphatic system from the interstitial spaces.
1. C14	White Blood Cells		2. Lymphocytes: White blood cells with clear cytoplasm and a single nucleus. Functions include recognition and destruction of bacteria, virus-infected cells, waste and foreign material.
2. L5	Lymph Nodes		
3. D1	Digestive System		

Notes:

Lymph System

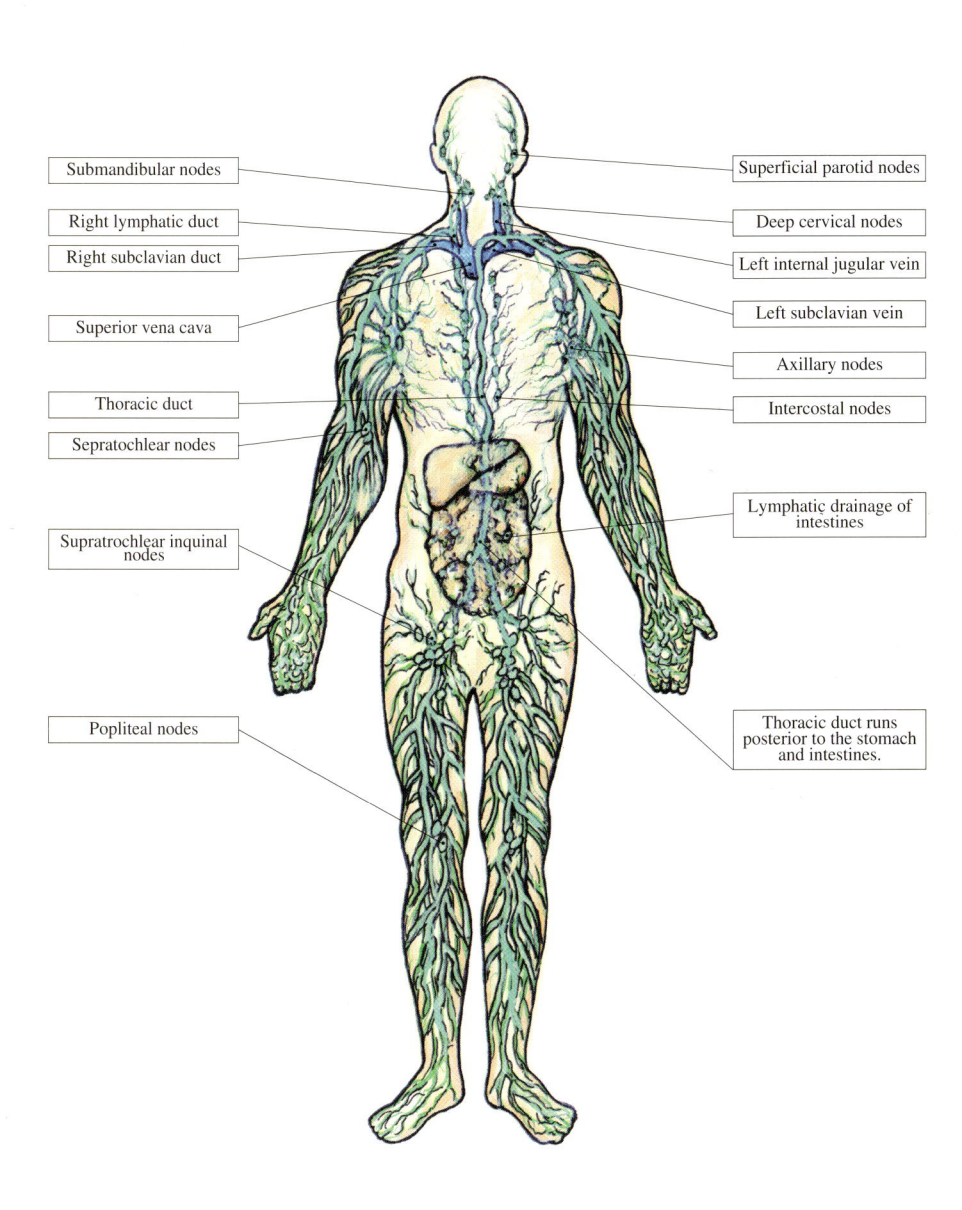

- Submandibular nodes
- Right lymphatic duct
- Right subclavian duct
- Superior vena cava
- Thoracic duct
- Sepratochlear nodes
- Supratrochlear inquinal nodes
- Popliteal nodes

- Superficial parotid nodes
- Deep cervical nodes
- Left internal jugular vein
- Left subclavian vein
- Axillary nodes
- Intercostal nodes
- Lymphatic drainage of intestines
- Thoracic duct runs posterior to the stomach and intestines.

Anterior view

L_1

Lymph
L_2

I. Location:
1. Present in the lymphatic vessels and nodes[1].

II. Structure:
1. Same composition as <u>interstitial</u> (intercellular) <u>fluid</u>. Both are almost identical to blood plasma[2], which is primarily water with some proteins. Lymph usually contains more waste products and cellular debris.

III. Function:
1. To serve as a medium for the transport of excess interstitial fluid and <u>plasma proteins</u> from the spaces between tissue cells back to the blood.

2. To carry waste products from cellular metabolism and debris from cellular damage or immune reactions to invaders from the interstitial space.

3. To act as a transport medium for absorbed fats and fat-soluble nutrients from the digestive tract to the blood.

Cross-Reference

Volume	Chapter
1	L1	Lymphatic System
2	C12	Composition of blood

Definitions
1. <u>Interstitial</u> (intercellular) <u>fluid</u>: The fluid found between the cells of the body.
2. <u>Plasma proteins</u>: Large protein molecules found in blood, plasma, interstitial fluid, and lymph. They serve a variety of functions throughout the body.

<u>Notes:</u>

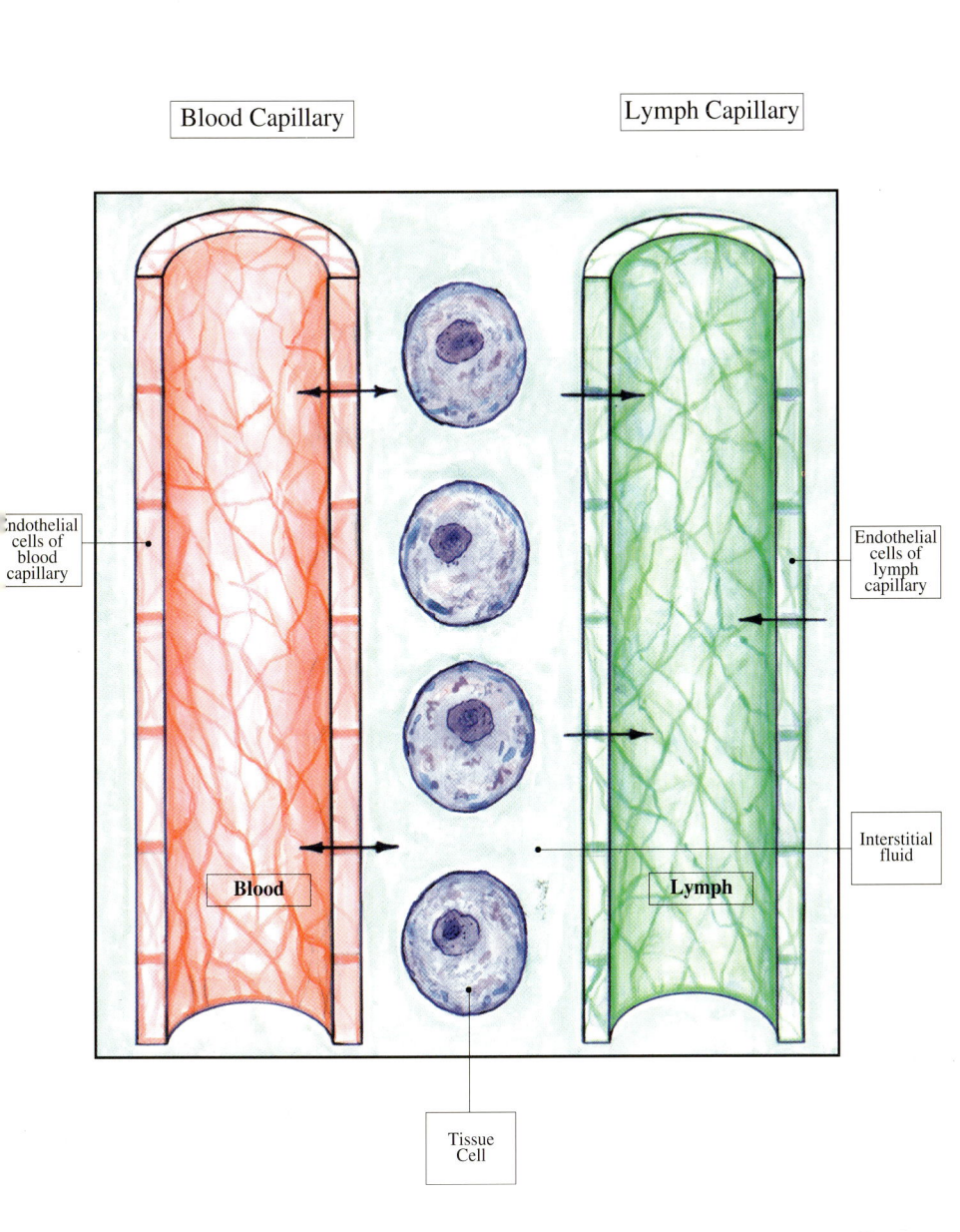

Lymph

Blood Capillary

Lymph Capillary

Endothelial cells of blood capillary

Endothelial cells of lymph capillary

Blood

Lymph

Interstitial fluid

Tissue Cell

Lymphatic Capillaries
L₃

I. Location:
   1. Present in most tissue except avascular structures (hair, nails, cornea, epidermis) and from central nervous tissue.

II. Structure:
   1. An extensive capillary network[1] consisting of minute tubules with a permeable endothelium[2] that is continuous with lymphatic vessels, thus forming a closed system.
   2. The junctions between the endothelial cells are often open though the edges of the cells may overlap. This arrangement allows fluid and proteins to enter but not leave the lymph capillaries.
   3. Color : yellowish or transparent.
   4. The number and size of capillary plexuses differ depending on the location.
   5. Where lymph capillaries are most abundant they are arranged in two or more anastomosing layers (a superficial and a deep layer).
   6. Lymph capillaries have an irregular shape.

III. Function:
   1. The extensive capillary network collects interstitial fluid[2] from various tissues and organs. Once inside the lymph vessels, this fluid is called lymph.
   2. The lymph system provides a drainage system for excess interstitial fluid and plasma proteins that have escaped from the blood.
   3. Lymph is then transported into lymphatic vessels[3], where it will be passed through filtering lymph nodes[4] before re-entering the bloodstream.
   4. Lymph capillaries absorb fat and fat-soluble nutrients from the digestive tract, and transport them to the blood[5].

Cross-Reference

Volume	Chapter
1	L1	Lymphatic System
2	L2	Lymph
3	L4	Lymphatic vessels
4	L5	Lymph Nodes
5	D1	Digestive System

Definitions
1. Endothelium: A membrane consisting of narrow, flattened cells which line lymph and blood vessels.
2. Plexus: Interbranching network of nerves, blood or lymph vessels.
3. Anastomosis: Connection between parts of any branching system as of blood or lymph system.

Notes:

Lymphatic Capillaries

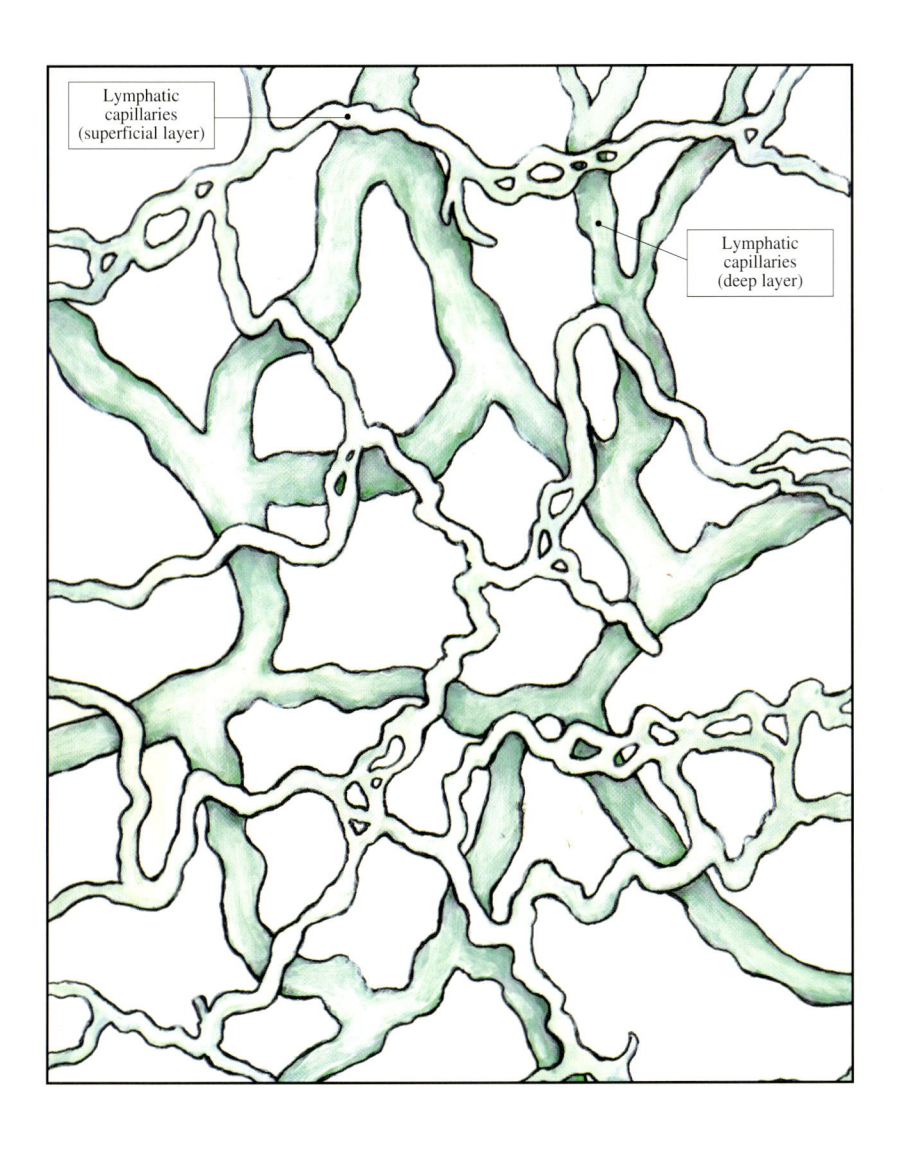

Lymphatic Vessels
L_4

I. Location:
1. Lymphatic vessels are formed by the emergence of lymph capillaries[1]. They therefore are found in or near all the vascular tissues of the body. The vessels ultimately unite to form two large vessels; The <u>thoracic</u> and the <u>right lymphatic ducts</u> that drain into the subclavian veins[2].

2. Lymphatics in the skin generally follow veins, while those of the viscera or internal organs generally follow arteries.

II. Structure:
1. Larger vessels have three layers similar to small veins, but have thinner walls and more valves[3].

2. The many valves give the lymphatic vessels a knotted or headed appearance.

3. Lymphatics pass through masses of lymph tissue called lymph nodes[4] at various intervals along their course.

4. Where abundant, they are arranged in a superficial and deep set.

III. Function:
1. To carry lymph from lymph capillaries through lymph nodes, waste can be filtered before re-entering the bloodstream.

2. To carry absorbed fats and fat-soluble nutrients to the blood for circulation.

3. To keep lymph flowing in the proper direction by the opening and closing of valves.

4. Though the valves help ensure a one way flow, the lymph system has no pump to force lymph through its vessels. Various factors provide the force for lymph flow: Including skeletal muscle contraction that "milks" the vessels, respiration-induced changes in thoracic pressure, the velocity of the blood in the veins into which the lymph vessels empty, and some due to the contraction of the smooth muscle in the walls of the lymphatics.

Cross-Reference

Volume	Chapter
1 L3	Lymphatic Capillaries
2 L1	Lymphatic System
3 C11	Veins
4 L5	Lymph Nodes

Definitions

1. <u>Thoracic duct</u>: Common trunk of all lymphatic vessels of the body except those of the upper right side of the body.
2. <u>Right Lymphatic Duct</u>: Common trunk of all lymphatic vessels of the right upper extremity and those of the right side of the head, neck and thorax.

<u>Notes</u>:

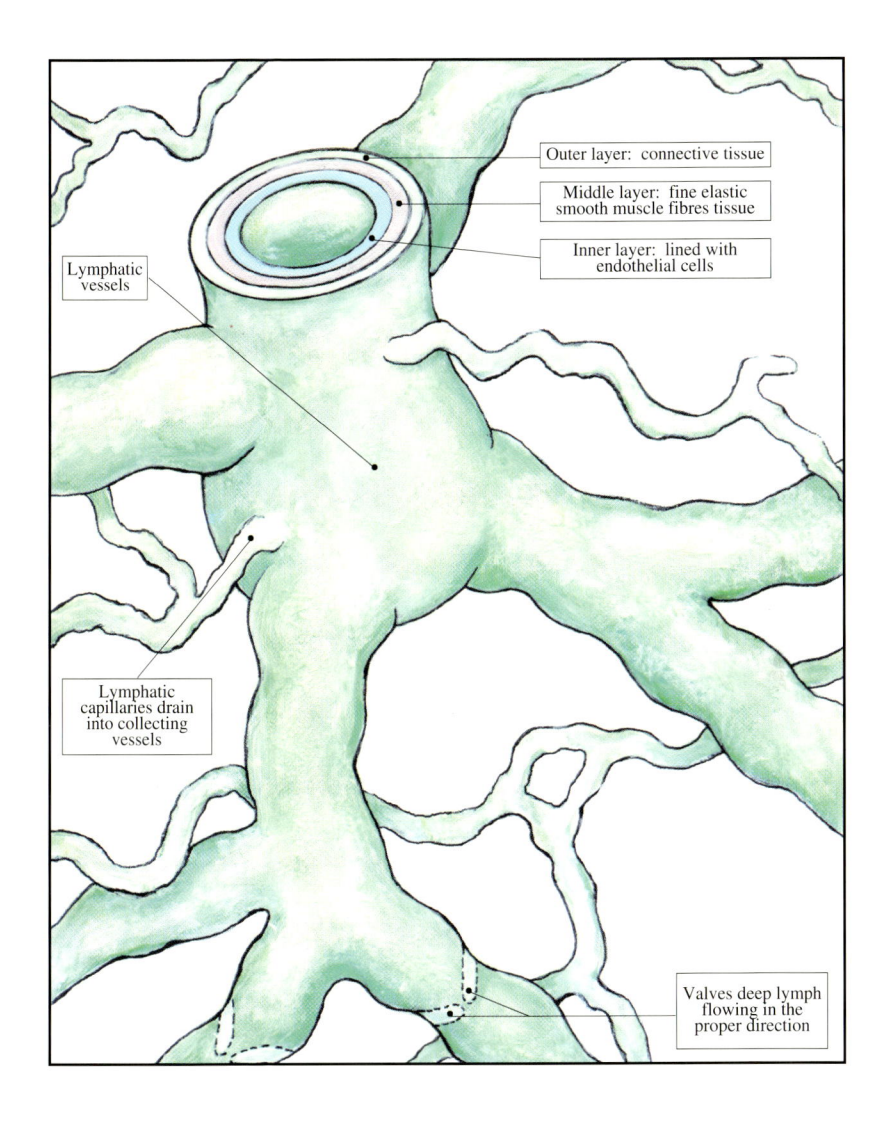

Lymphatic Vessels

- Outer layer: connective tissue
- Middle layer: fine elastic smooth muscle fibres tissue
- Inner layer: lined with endothelial cells
- Lymphatic vessels
- Lymphatic capillaries drain into collecting vessels
- Valves deep lymph flowing in the proper direction

L_4

Lymph Nodes
L$_5$

I. Location:
1. Interspersed along the length of lymphatic vessels, with large masses commonly located at the neck, ear, underarm, groin, knees and between ribs[1].

II. Structure:
1. Small oval-shaped bodies in the course of lymphatic vessels, ranging in size from 1-25 mm (0.04-1") in length.

2. Slight indentation on one side, the hilum through which some lymph vessels leave.

3. Lymph enters the node through afferent vessels, and leaves through efferent vessels.

4. Differing cell zones are all encased in the collagen and elastin fiber of the capsule, with extensions of this capsule (trabeculae) dividing the node into the zones.

5. Each cell zone has differing amounts of lymphocytes and macrophages[2].

III. Function:
1. Through phagocytosis, the lymphocytes and macrophages in the lymph nodes trap and digest waste matter, dead cells and bacteria.

2. Like other lymph tissue, lymphocytes which will attack bacteria and waste by recognizing previous antigens through "immunological memory". In addition, some lymphocytes will add proteins in the form of antibodies to blood.

3. Infected lymph nodes can become enlarged and tender during illness or by an infection in the region drained by lymphatics that pass through the nodes.

Cross-Reference

Volume	Chapter
1 L1	Lymphatic System
2 C14	White Blood Cells

Notes:

Definitions
1. Phagocytosis: The ingestion and destruction by phagocytes of cells, microorganisms, etc.
2. Antigen: An enzyme, toxin or other substance, usually of high molecular weight, to which the body reacts by producing antibodies.
3. Antibody: A protein produced in the body in response to contact of the body with an antigen, and having the specific capacity of neutralizing, hence creating immunity to the antigen.

Lymph Nodes

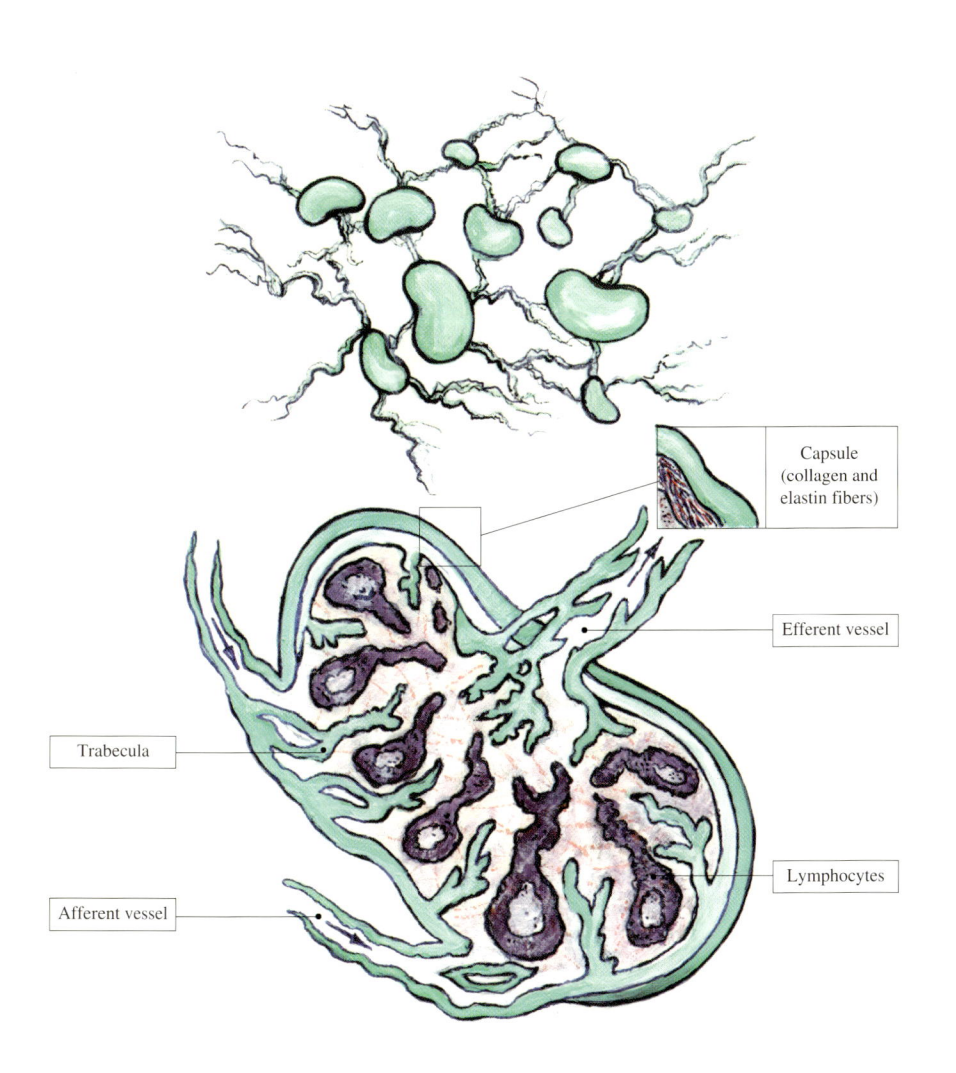

Note: Arrows show direction of lymph flow.

Palatine and Lingual Tonsils
L_6

I. Location:
1. Lingual tonsil is embedded in submucosa, in the pharyngeal part or base of the tongue.
2. Palatine tonsils are located in the posterior walls of the pharynx[1].
3. Each palatine tonsil lies between the palatoglossal and palatopharyngeal arches.

II. Structure:
1. Lymph tissue encapsulated in a mucous membrane.
2. Tonsillar lymphoid tissue is arranged in nodules of follicles[2], where lymphocytes and macrophages are massed.

III. Function:
1. To provide humoral and cellular defense against infection of the oral and nasal cavities, by storing and/or producing lymphocytes and macrophages.
2. Palatine tonsils are those most commonly removed by a tonsillectomy.

Cross-Reference

Volume	Chapter
1. D8	Pharynx
2. L5	Lymph nodes

Definitions
1. Pharynx: Muscle and membranous cavity of alimentary canal leading from the mouth and nasal passages to the larynx and esophagus.
2. Humoral: Pertaining to fluids of the body.

Notes:

Palatine and Lingual Tonsils

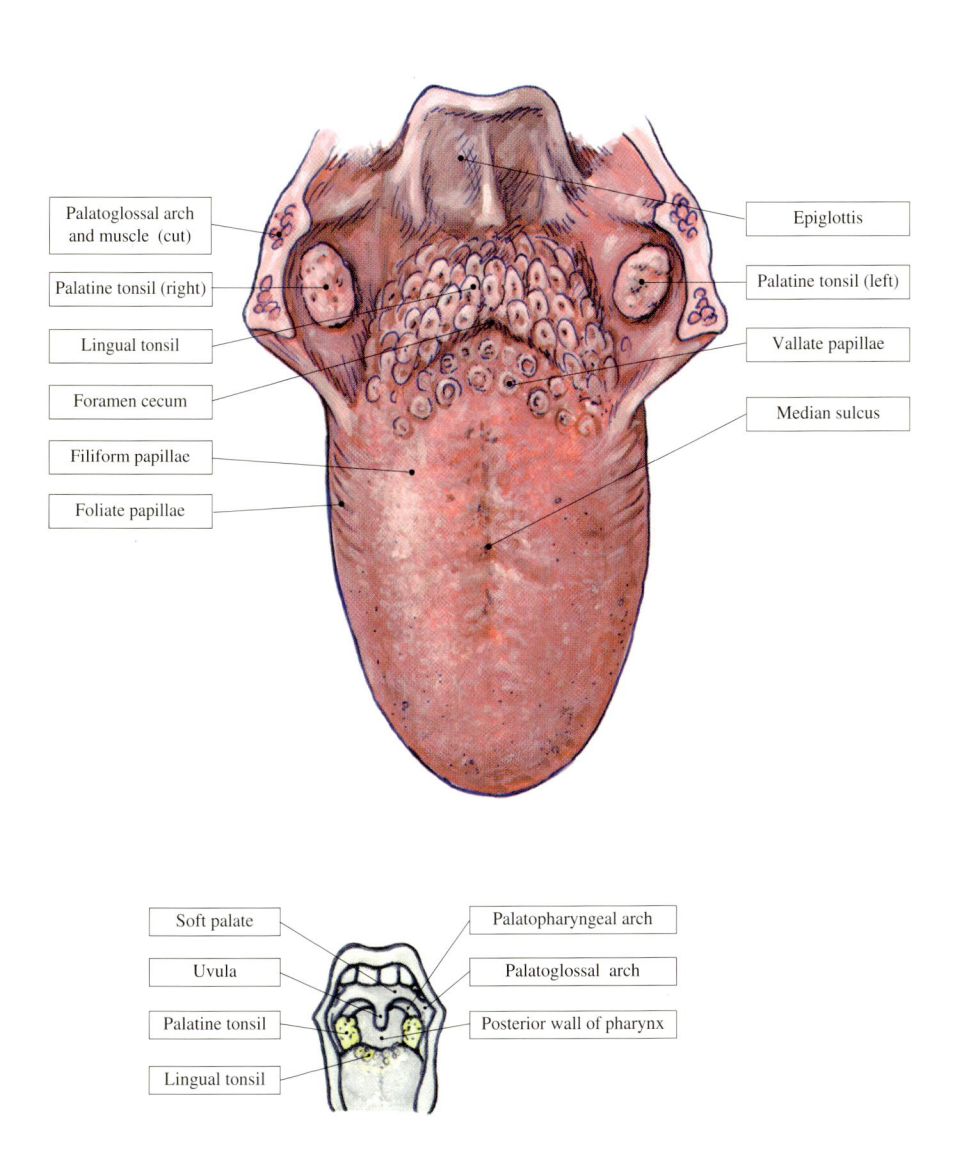

Palatoglossal arch and muscle (cut)	Epiglottis
Palatine tonsil (right)	Palatine tonsil (left)
Lingual tonsil	Vallate papillae
Foramen cecum	Median sulcus
Filiform papillae	
Foliate papillae	

Soft palate	Palatopharyngeal arch
Uvula	Palatoglossal arch
Palatine tonsil	Posterior wall of pharynx
Lingual tonsil	

Pharyngeal Tonsil
L₇

I. Location:
1. It is posterior and superior (behind and above) to the palatine and lingual tonsils[1].
2. Its <u>apex</u> is at the <u>nasal septum</u>, and it's base is at the junction of the nasopharyngeal roof and posterior wall.

II. Structure:
1. Lymphatic tissue encapsulated in a mucous membrane.
2. Not visible until later fetal months.
3. Begins to diminish in size after six to seven years.

III. Function:
1. Guards the pharynx from infection by producing and/or storing lymphocytes and macrophages.
2. When infected, they become swollen and are referred to as the <u>adenoids</u>, which can interfere with breathing and speech.

Cross-Reference
Volume	Chapter
1	L6 — Palatine and Lingual Tonsil

Definitions
1. <u>Apex</u>: The highest point, peak, vertex.
2. <u>Nasal septum</u>: Divides the nasal passage in two, left and right.
3. <u>Adenoids</u>: Swollen growths of lymphoid tissue in the upper part of the throat, can obstruct breathing and sleeping.

<u>Notes</u>:

Pharyngeal Tonsil

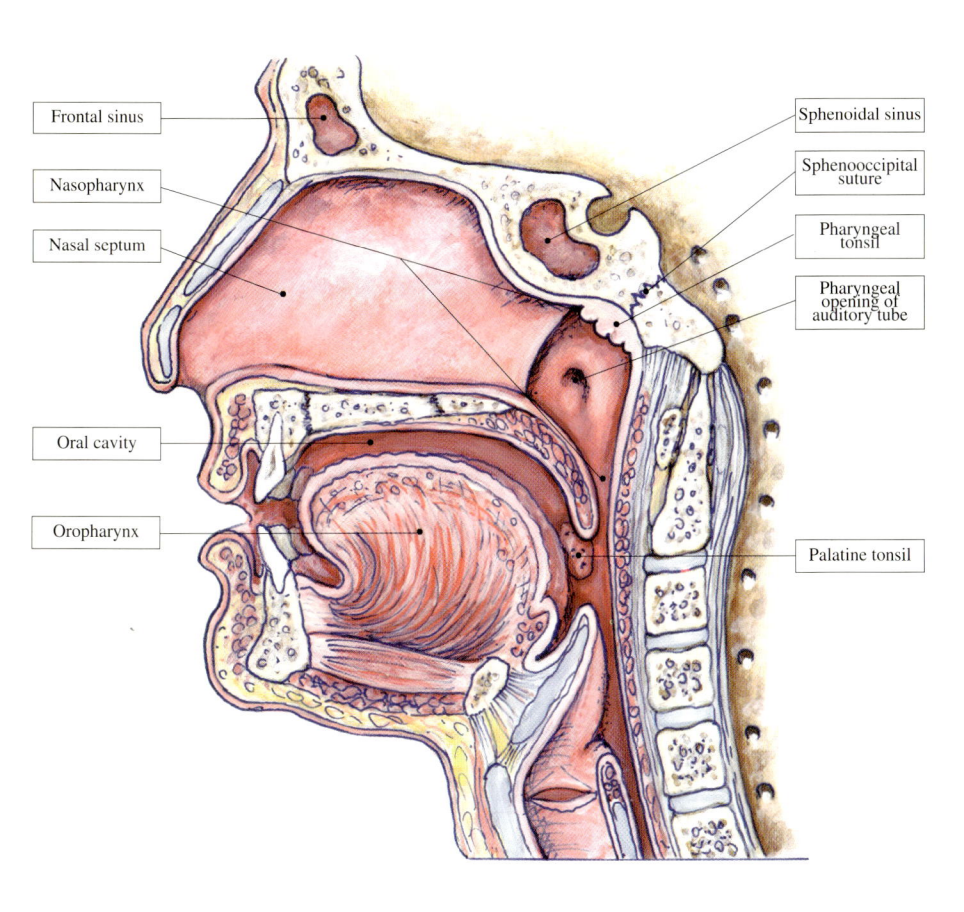

Peyer's Patches
L_8

I. Location:
1. Can be found in the walls of <u>alimentary tracts</u>[1], usually in the small intestine[2].
2. Due to location, Peyer's Patches are known as gut-associated lymphoid tissue (GALT).

II. Structure:
1. Consists of <u>aggregated</u> lymphatic tissue or nodules.

III. Function:
1. To provide and store lymphocytes and/or macrophages in the alimentary tract.

Cross-Reference

Volume	Chapter
1. D1	Digestive System
2. D16	Small Intestine

Definitions
1. <u>Alimentary tract</u>: Tube and its enlargements through which food passes and in which it is digested extending from mouth thru esophagus, stomach, intestines, and anus.
2. <u>Aggregated</u>: Gathered into or considered as a whole.

Notes:

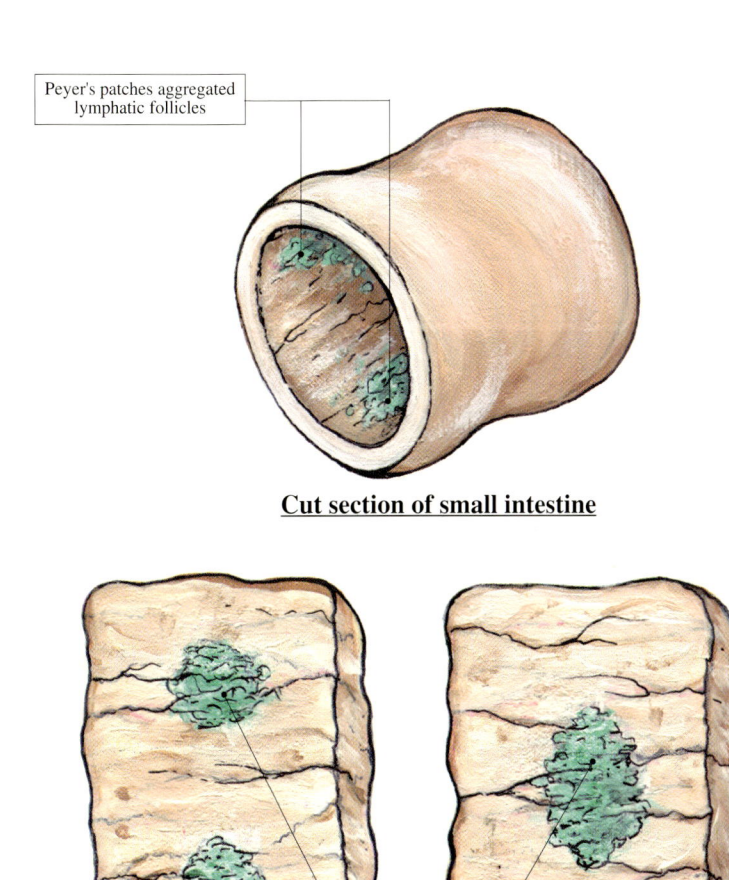

Peyer's Patches

Peyer's patches aggregated lymphatic follicles

Cut section of small intestine

A *B*

Peyer's patches in the (A)proximal and (B)distal parts of the intestine

L_8

Spleen
L_9

I. Location:
1. The spleen is located in the upper left (hypochondriac) region of the abdomen.

2. It is bordered on its lower anterior surface by the transverse and descending colon (colic); on its upper anterior surface by the stomach (gastric); on its medial border by the left kidney (renal); and on its upper posterior surface by the diaphragm.

II. Structure:
1. Size:
   - Birth - approx. 2 cm. length, 1 cm. breadth, 1/4 cm. thick, weight approx. 17 gram.
   - Adult - approx. 12 cm. length, 7 cm. breadth, 3-4 cm. thick, weight approx. 150 gram.

2. Two coats: outer serous layer and internal fibrous capsule, which sends branching trabeculae into interior.

3. The inner surface contains two different kinds of tissue, white and red pulp. White pulp is essentially lymph tissue, where as the red pulp is sinuses filled with blood.

4. The splenic artery and vein enter the spleen through the hilus.

III. Function:
1. The spleen phagocytizes bacteria, worn-out red blood cells, and debris from the blood[1].

2. The spleen produces lymphocytes and plasma cells to be exchanged with the blood.

3. Stores some red blood cells for release into the blood, if needed.

4. A damaged spleen can be removed and its functions assumed by other organs.

Cross-Reference
Volume	Chapter
1. L5	Lymph Nodes

Definitions
1. Hilus: A small recess or opening where veins and/or nerves enter an organ.
2. Plasma cells: An activated type of lymphocyte that produces antibodies.

Notes:

Spleen

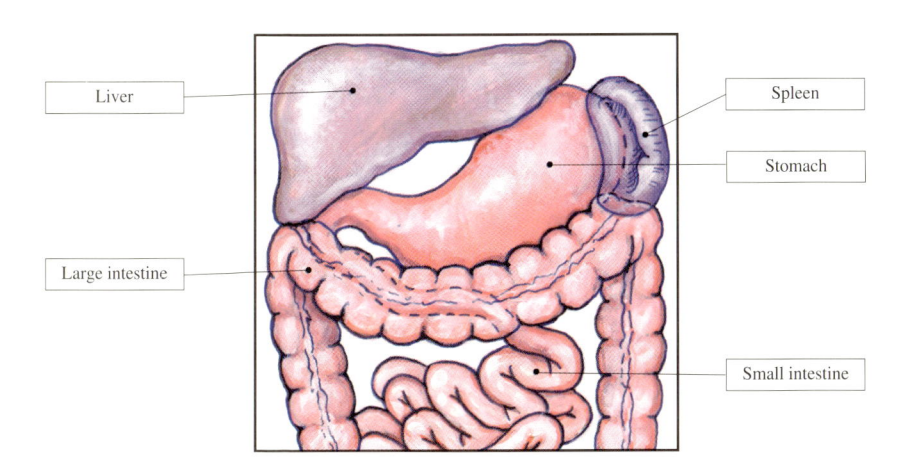

Anterior view

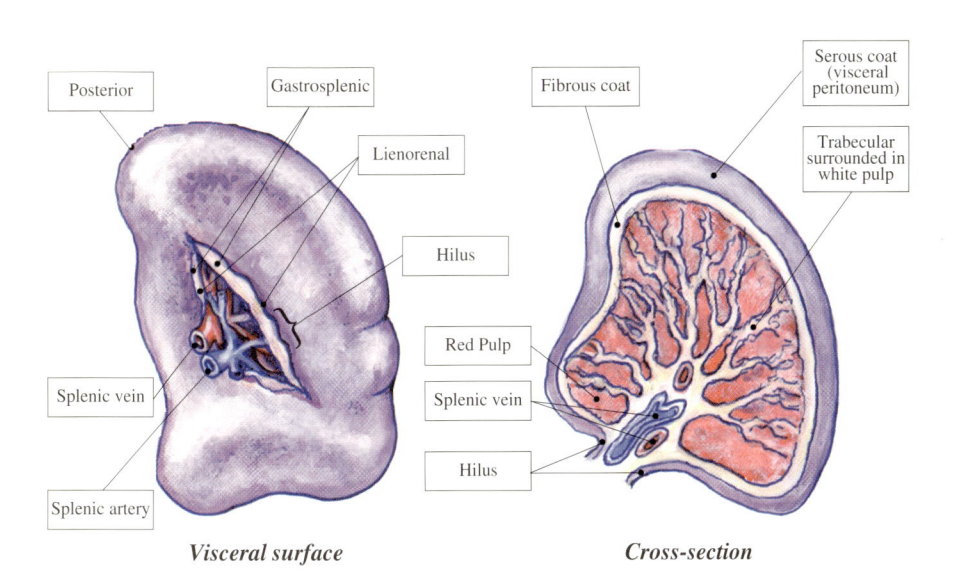

Visceral surface *Cross-section*

Anterior view

Thymus
L[10]

I. Location:
1. Occupies the upper anterior part of the thorax[1].

2. Anterior: <u>sternum</u>, sternohyoid, and sternothyroid muscles.

3. Posterior are the <u>pericardium</u>[2], the aortic arches, and the front and sides of the trachea[3].

II. Structure:
1. Varies in size and activity depending on the age, disease, and the physiological state of the body.

2. Weight:
   Birth: 10-15 gram.
   Puberty: 30-40 gram, then diminishes with old age and is largely replaced by fat.

3. Consists of two unequal pyramidal lobes.

4. Each lobe consists of a loose fibrous capsule, a highly cellular cortex, and a less dense medulla containing lymphocytes and macrophages.

5. Many of these same cells are found in the interlobular connective tissue.

6. Color:
   Birth: Pinkish-grey.
   Adult: yellowish (due to replacement by fat).

III. Function:
1. Process immature lymphocytes from the bone marrow into T-lymphocytes (T-cells), which help in immune responses[4].

2. Produce the hormone thymosin, which plays a role in developing other immature lymphocytes into B lymphocytes (B-cells), which help in immune responses[4].

Cross-Reference

Volume	Chapter
1 C3	Structure of the Heart
2 C2.5	Pericardium and Heart Walls
3 R5	Trachea
4. L1	Lymph System

Definitions
1. <u>Sternum</u>: The flat bone running down the center of the chest and connected to the ribs.
2. <u>Pericardium</u>: Thin membranous sac surrounding the heart and the roots of the great vessels.

<u>Notes</u>:

Thymus

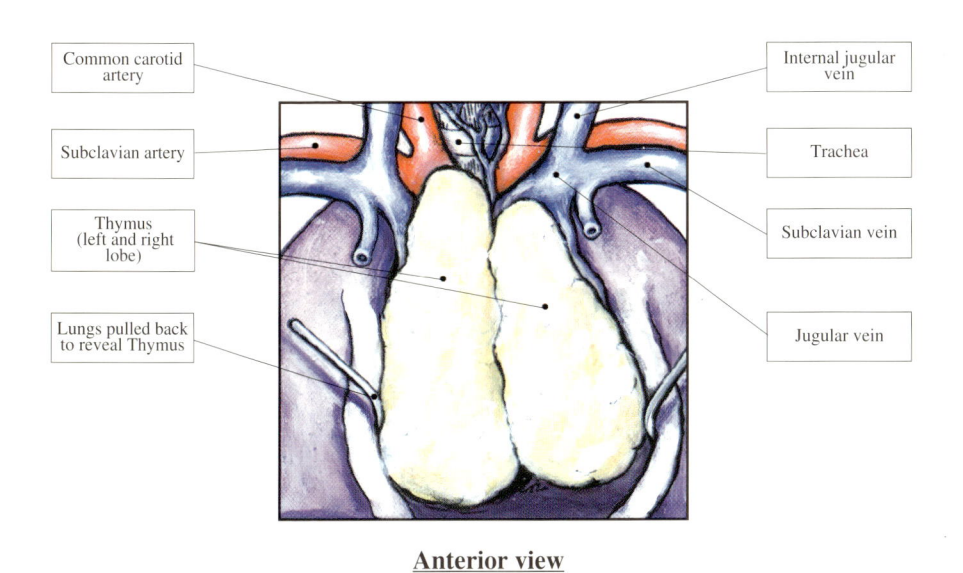

Common carotid artery	Internal jugular vein
Subclavian artery	Trachea
Thymus (left and right lobe)	Subclavian vein
Lungs pulled back to reveal Thymus	Jugular vein

Anterior view

Capsule	Medulla
Cortex	Interlobular connective tissue

Cross-section of thymus

L_{10}

Lymph System

Identification
(Match the letter with the term)

___ Deep Cervical nodes

___ Intercostal nodes

___ Superior vena cava

___ Supratrochlear inquinal nodes

___ Superficial parotid nodes

___ Sepratochlear nodes

___ Right lymphatic duct

___ Thoracic duct

___ Left internal jugular vein

___ Lymphatic drainage of intestines

___ Right Subclavian duct

___ Left subclavian vein

___ Submandibular nodes

___ Axillary nodes

___ Popliteal nodes

___ Thoracic duct runs posterior to the stomach and intestines

Questions
(Fill in the bank with the appropriate answer)

1. _____ remove the debris, and cellular waste, by the process of _____.

2. Fluid collected by the lymphatic system from the interstitial space is called _____.

3. The lymphatic system is essential to the body's _____, it has the ability to destroy invading bacteria and remove dead and damaged tissue.

4. Lymphoid _____ store, process or produce.

5. Name the seven Lymphoid tissues:

   _____   _____

   _____   _____

   _____   _____

   _____

Lymph System

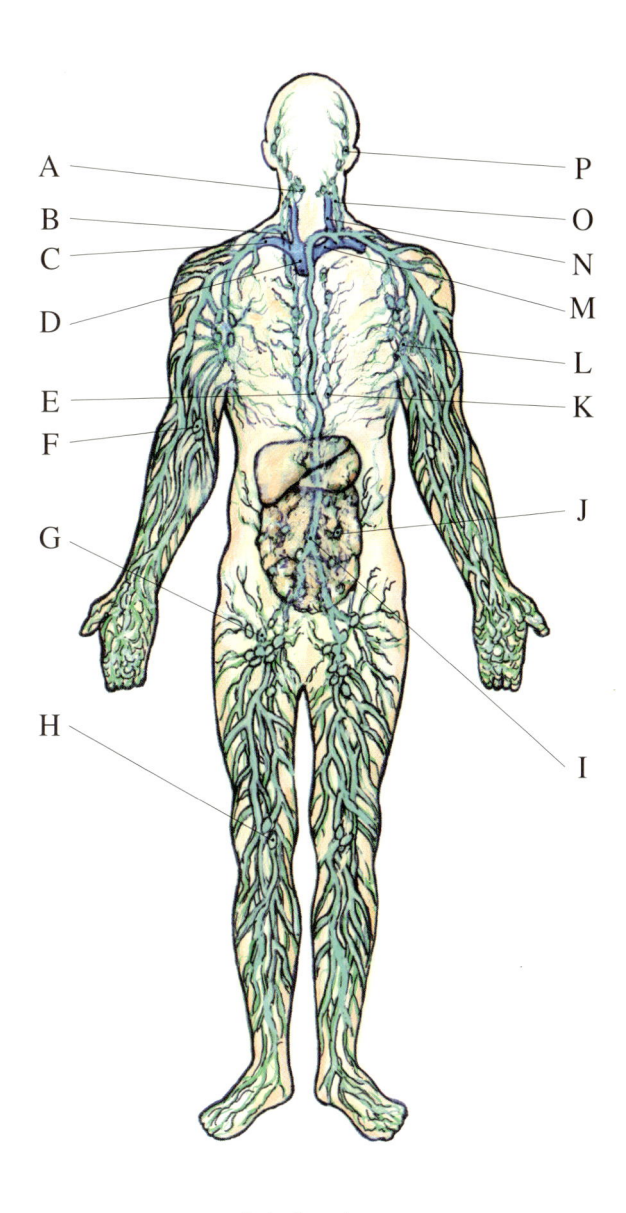

Anterior view

Lymph

Identification
(Match the letter with the term)

___ Tissue Cell   ___ Endothelial cells of lymph capillary

___ Interstitial fluid   ___ Endothelial cells of blood capillary

Questions
(Fill in the blank with the appropriate answer)

1. Lymph acts as a transport medium for _____ and _____ from the digestive tract to the blood.

2. Lymph serves as a medium for the transport of excess _____ and _____ from the spaces between tissue cells back to the blood.

3. Lymph is present in the _____ and _____.

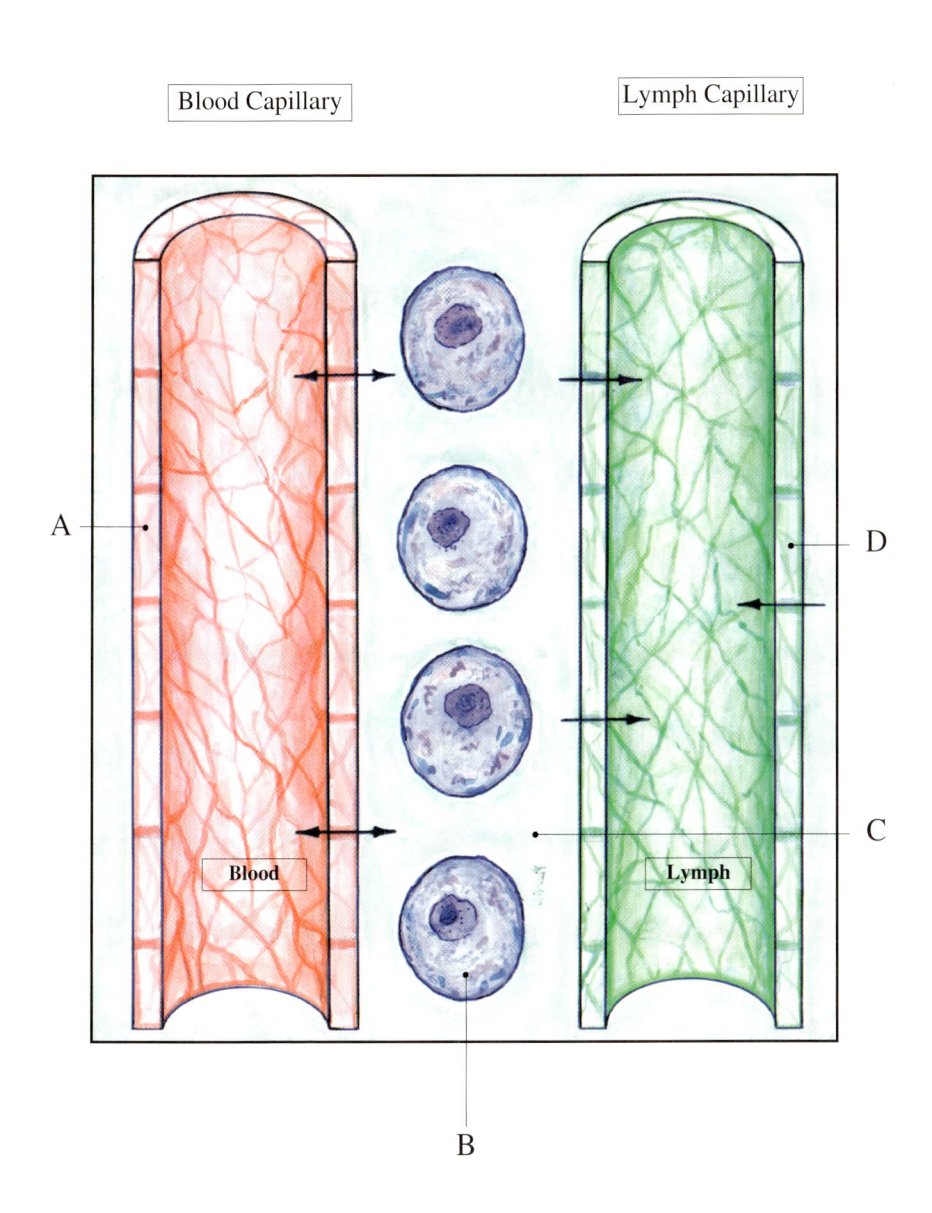

Lymph

Blood Capillary

Lymph Capillary

A

Blood

B

C

Lymph

D

Lymphatic Capillaries

Identification
(Match the letter with the term)

___ Lymphatic capillaries (superficial layer)

___ Lymphatic capillaries (deep layer)

Questions
(Fill in the blank with the appropriate answer)

1. The lymph system provides a drainage system for excess _____ and _____ that have escaped from the blood.

2. Connection between parts of any branching system as of blood or lymph system is called _____.

3. The number and size of capillary _____ differ depending on the location.

4. A membrane consisting of narrow, flattened cells, which line lymph and blood vessels is called _____.

Lymphatic Capillaries

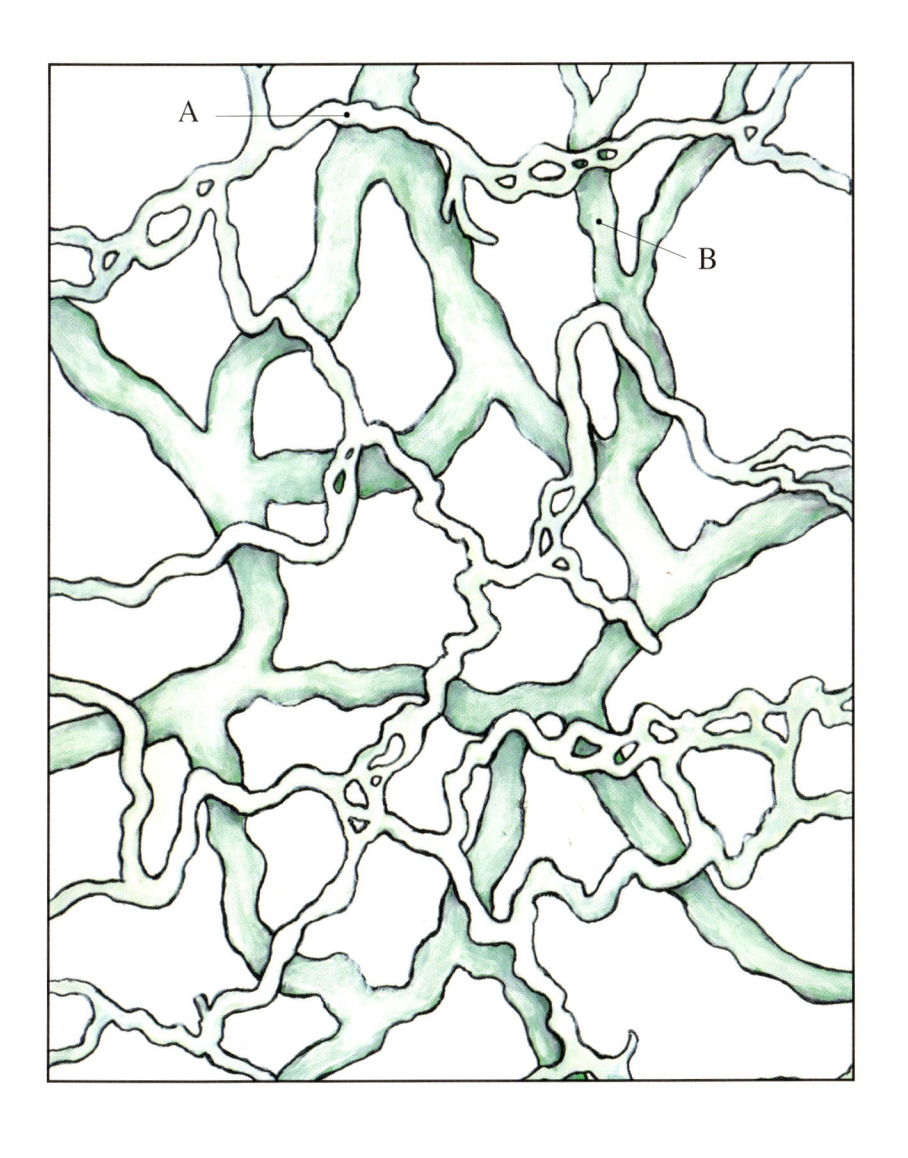

Lymphatic Vessels

Identification
(Match the letter with the term)

___ Inner layer: fine elastic smooth muscle fibrous tissue

___ Valves deep lymph flowing in the proper direction

___ Lymphatic vessels

___ Outer layer: connective tissue

___ Lymphatic capillaries drain into collecting vessels

___ Middle layer: fine elastic smooth muscle fibrous tissue

Questions
(Fill in the blank with the appropriate answer)

1. The _____ is the common trunk of all lymphatic vessels of the body except those of the upper right side of the body.

2. Lymphatics pass through masses of lymph tissue called _____, at various intervals along their course.

3. Lymphatic _____ are formed by the the emergence of lymph _____.

4. The _____ is the common trunk of all lymphatic vessels of the right upper extremity and those of the right side of the head, neck, and thorax.

Lymphatic Vessels

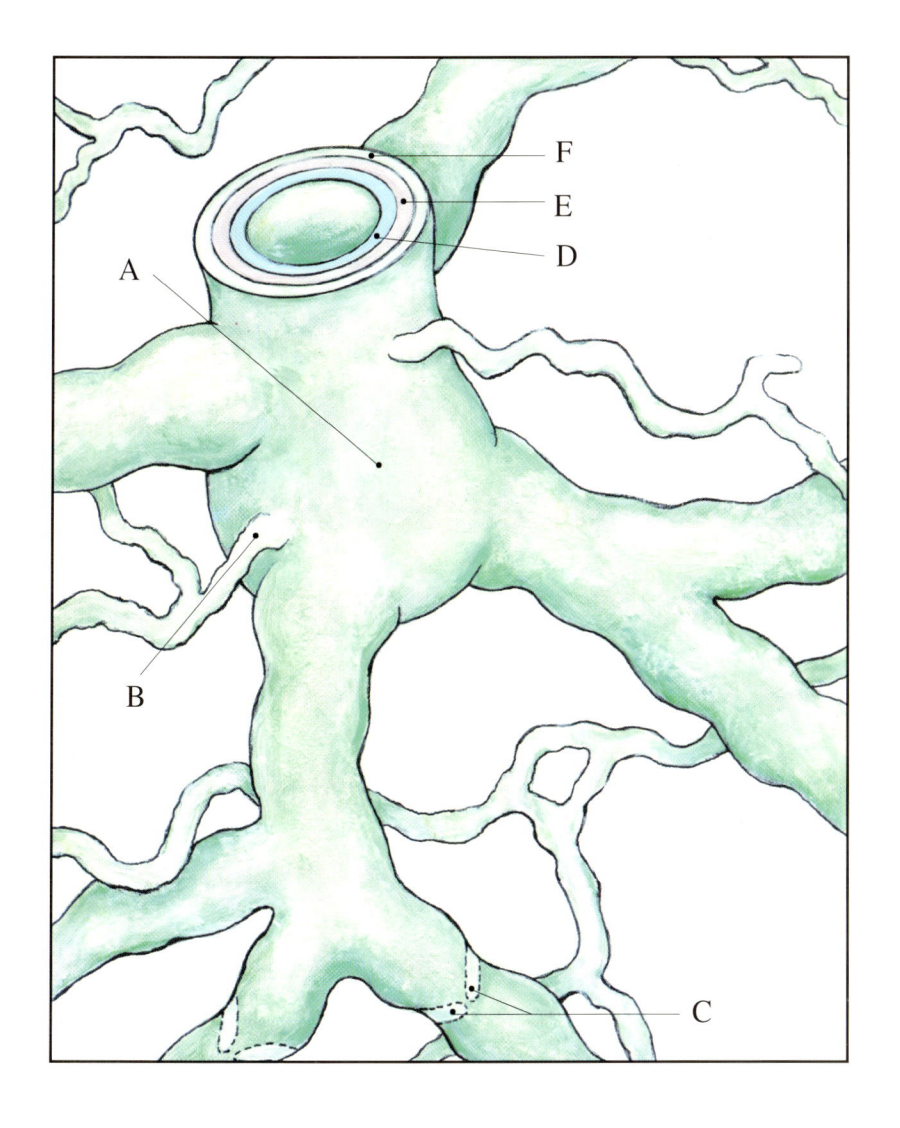

Lymph Nodes

Identification
(Match the letter with the term)

___ Efferent vessel

___ Trabecula

___ Afferent vessel

___ Capsule (collagen and elastin fibres)

___ Lymphocytes

Questions
(Fill in the blank with the appropriate answer)

1. Like other lymph tissue, lymphocytes which will attack bacteria and waste, by recognizing previous _____ through "immunological memory" In addition, some lymphocytes will add proteins in the form of _____ to blood.

2. Through _____, the lymphocytes and macrophages in the lymph nodes trap and digest waste matter, dead cells, and bacteria.

3. Lymph enter the node through _____, and leaves through _____.

4. Each cell zone has differing amounts of _____ and _____.

Lymph Nodes

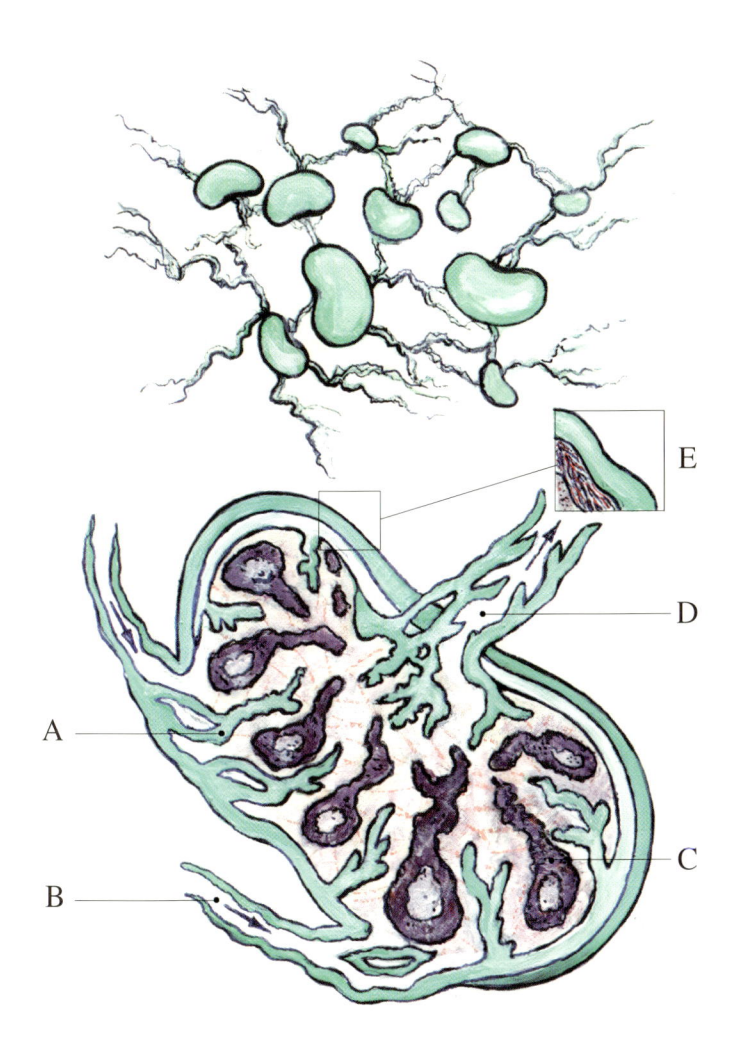

Note: Arrows show direction of lymph flow.

Palatine and Lingual Tonsils

Identification
(Match the letter with the term)

___ Vallate papillae

___ Palatoglossal arch

___ Foramen cecum

___ Lingual tonsil

___ Uvula

___ Filiform papillae

___ Epiglottis

___ Foliate papillae

___ Posterior wall of pharynx

___ Palatine tonsil (left)

___ Median sulcus

___ Palatopharyngeal arch

___ Soft palate

___ Palatine tonsil (right)

___ Lingual tonsil

___ Palatoglossal arch and muscle (cut)

___ Palatine tonsil

Questions
(Fill in the blank with the appropriate answer)

1. To provide _____ and cellular defense against infection of the oral and nasal cavities, by storing and/or producing lymphocytes and macrophages.

2. The _____ is embedded in submucosa in the pharyngeal part or base of the tongue.

3. The _____ are located in the posterior walls of the pharynx.

4. Each Palatine tonsil lies between the _____ and _____.

Palatine and Lingual Tonsils

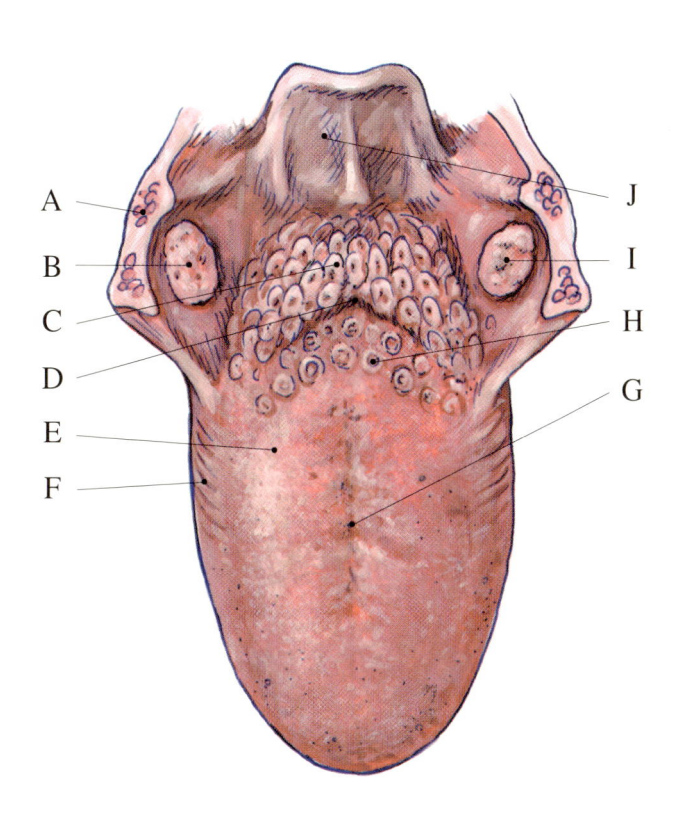

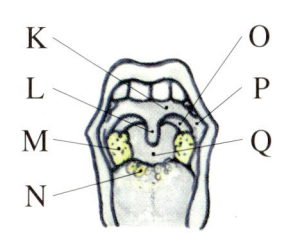

Pharyngeal Tonsil

Identification
(Match the letter with the term)

___ Palatine tonsil

___ Pharyngeal tonsil

___ Nasopharynx

___ Sphenooccipital suture

___ Oral cavity

___ Frontal sinus

___ Nasal septum

___ Oropharynx

___ Sphenoidal sinus

___ Pharyngeal opening of auditory tube

Questions
(Fill in the blank with the appropriate answer)

1. After six to seven years _____ begin to diminish in size.

2. The Pharyngeal tonsil is _____ and superior to the palatine and _____ tonsils.

3. The _____ divides the nasal passages in two, left and right.

Pharyngeal Tonsil

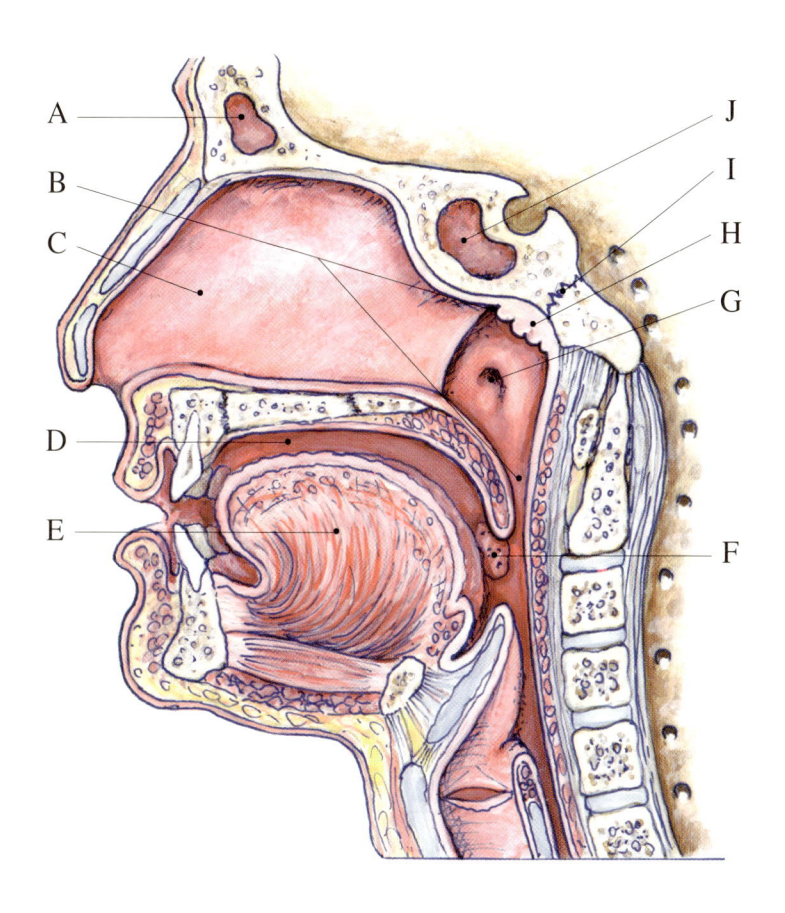

A

B

C

D

E

J

I

H

G

F

Peyer's Patches

Identification
(Match the letter with the term)

___ Peyer's patches in the (A) proximal and (B) distal parts of the intestine

___ Peyer's patches aggregated lymphatic follicles

Questions
(Fill in the blank with the appropriate answer)

1. Peyer's patches are known as gut-associated lymphoid tissue because of _____.

2. Peyer's patches can be found in the the walls of the _____.

3. The function of Peyer's patches are to provide and store _____ and _____.

Peyer's Patches

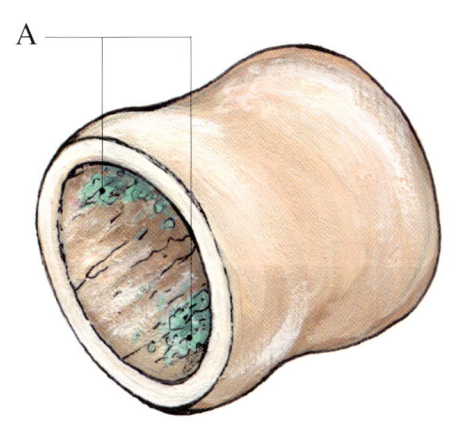

Cut section of small intestine

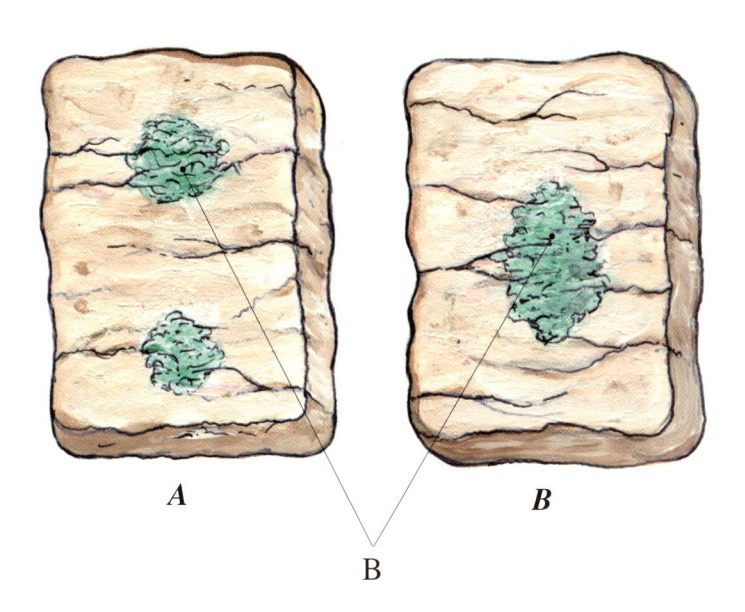

A *B*

Spleen

Identification
(Match the letter with the term)

___ Small intestine

___ Posterior extremity

___ Spleen

___ Serous coat (visceral peritoneum)

___ Hilus

___ Splenic vein

___ Stomach

___ Large intestine

___ Lienorenal ligament

___ Trabecular surrounded in white pulp

___ Fibrous coat (capsule)

___ Splenic vein and artery

___ Gastrosplenic ligament

___ Liver

___ Red pulp

___ Hilus

___ Splenic artery

Questions
(Fill in the blank with the appropriate answer)

1. The _____ is located in the upper left region of the abdomen.
2. The spleen produces _____ and _____ to be exchanged with the blood.
3. _____ and _____ enter the spleen through the hilus.
4. Functions can be assumed by other organs if _____ is damaged.
5. An activated type of lymphocyte that produces antibodies are _____.

Spleen

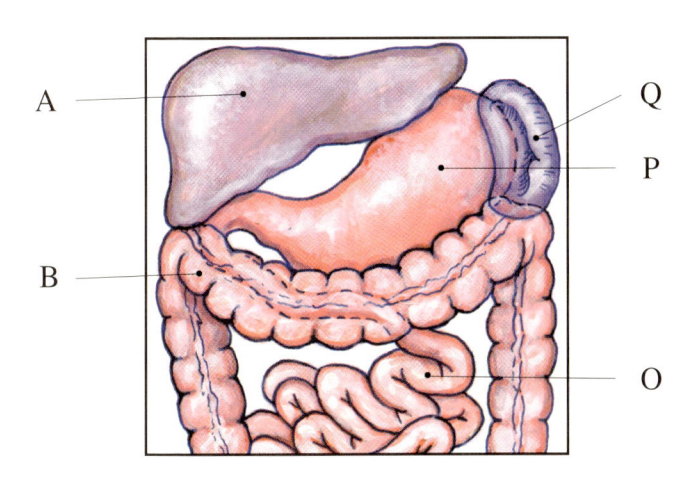

Anterior view

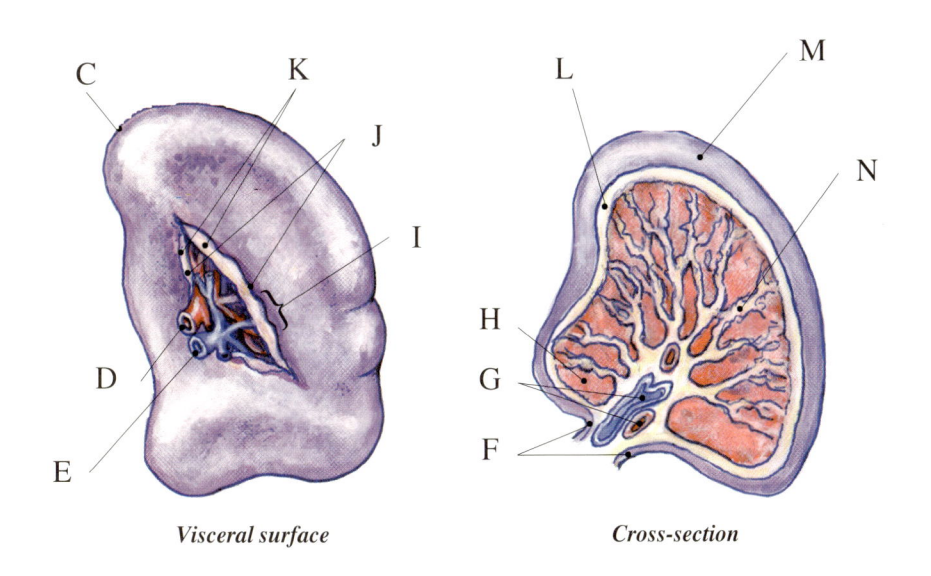

Visceral surface

Cross-section

Anterior view

Thymus

Identification
(Match the letter with the term)

___ Cortex

___ Trachea

___ Common carotid artery

___ Interlobular connective tissue

___ Jugular vein

___ Subclavian artery

___ Thymus (left and right lobe)

___ Capsule

___ Subclavian vein

___ Lungs pulled back to reveal Thymus

___ Medulla

___ Internal jugular vein

Questions
(Fill in the blank with the appropriate answer)

1. The thymus occupies the _____ part of the thorax.

2. The thymus consists of _____ unequal _____ lobes.

3. Many of the same cells are found in _____ tissue.

4. The thymus varies in size and activity depending on physiological,_____,and _____.

5. The _____ is the sac surrounding the heart and the roots of the great vessels.

Thymus

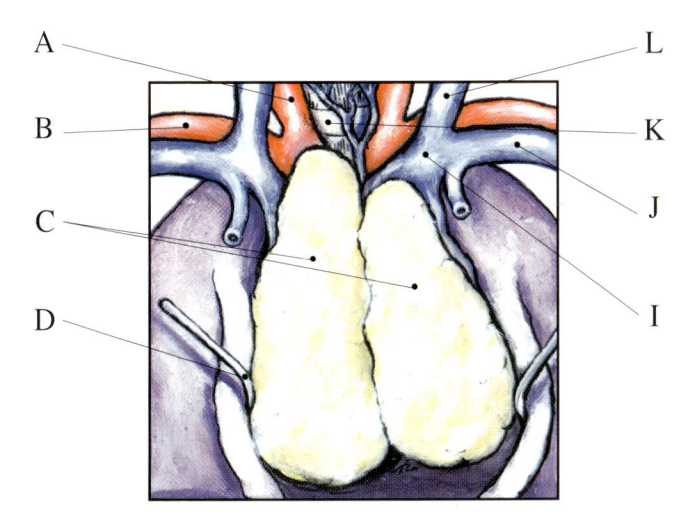

Anterior view

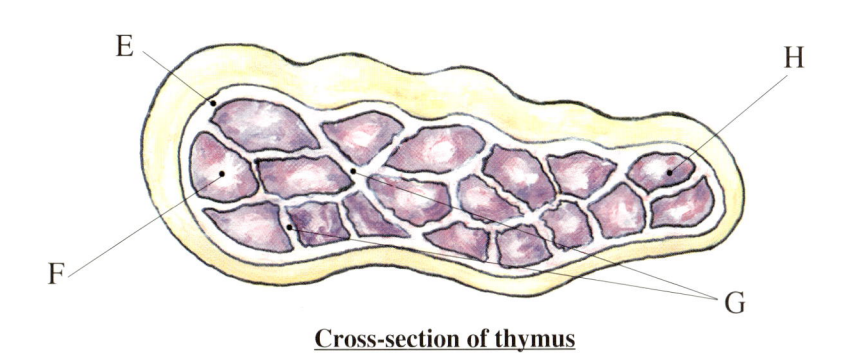

Cross-section of thymus

Address All Orders
or
Editorial Correspondence

to

Bryan Edwards Publishing Corporation
1284 E. Katella Avenue
Anaheim, California 92805

(800) 222-1775
or
(714) 634-0264

Printed on Recycled Paper

ISBN
1-878-576-26-7

CARDIOVASCULAR
HEART, VEINS, ARTERIES

LYMPHATIC
SPLEEN, THYMUS, LYMPH NODES

DIGESTIVE
STOMACH, INTESTINES, MOUTH

NERVOUS
BRAIN, SPINAL CORD

SPECIAL SENSES
SMELL, TASTE, SIGHT, HEARING, TOUCH

INTEGUMENT
HAIR, SKIN, NAILS

RESPIRATORY
LUNGS, THROAT, AIR PASSAGES

REPRODUCTIVE
GENITAL ORGANS

URINARY
KIDNEYS, URETERS, BLADDER

ENDOCRINE
DUCTLESS GLANDS

ISBN 1-878-576-32-1

Printed on Recycled Paper.